# Strain

Grower

Acquired $



| Indica | Hybrid | Sativa |
|---|---|---|

☐ Flower    ☐ Edible    ☐ Concentrate

## Symptoms Relieved



## Notes

| Effects | Strength | | | | |
|---|---|---|---|---|---|
| Peaceful | ○ | ○ | ○ | ○ | ○ |
| Sleepy | ○ | ○ | ○ | ○ | ○ |
| Pain Relief | ○ | ○ | ○ | ○ | ○ |
| Hungry | ○ | ○ | ○ | ○ | ○ |
| Uplifted | ○ | ○ | ○ | ○ | ○ |
| Creative | ○ | ○ | ○ | ○ | ○ |

**Ratings** ☆ ☆ ☆ ☆ ☆

# Strain

Grower

Date

Acquired

$

| Indica | Hybrid | Sativa |

☐ Flower  ☐ Edible  ☐ Concentrate

## Symptoms Relieved

## Notes



| Effects | Strength |
| --- | --- |
| Peaceful | ○ ○ ○ ○ ○ |
| Sleepy | ○ ○ ○ ○ ○ |
| Pain Relief | ○ ○ ○ ○ ○ |
| Hungry | ○ ○ ○ ○ ○ |
| Uplifted | ○ ○ ○ ○ ○ |
| Creative | ○ ○ ○ ○ ○ |

**Ratings** ☆ ☆ ☆ ☆ ☆

# Strain

Grower

Date

Acquired

$

| Indica | Hybrid | Sativa |

☐ Flower   ☐ Edible   ☐ Concentrate

## Symptoms Relieved

## Notes



| Effects | Strength |
|---------|----------|
| Peaceful | ○ ○ ○ ○ ○ |
| Sleepy | ○ ○ ○ ○ ○ |
| Pain Relief | ○ ○ ○ ○ ○ |
| Hungry | ○ ○ ○ ○ ○ |
| Uplifted | ○ ○ ○ ○ ○ |
| Creative | ○ ○ ○ ○ ○ |

**Ratings** ☆ ☆ ☆ ☆ ☆

# Strain

Grower

Date

Acquired

$

| Indica | Hybrid | Sativa |

☐ Flower   ☐ Edible   ☐ Concentrate

## Symptoms Relieved

Sweet
Fruity
Floral
Sour
Spicy
Earthy
Herbal
Woodsy

## Notes

| Effects | Strength | | | | |
| --- | --- | --- | --- | --- | --- |
| Peaceful | ○ | ○ | ○ | ○ | ○ |
| Sleepy | ○ | ○ | ○ | ○ | ○ |
| Pain Relief | ○ | ○ | ○ | ○ | ○ |
| Hungry | ○ | ○ | ○ | ○ | ○ |
| Uplifted | ○ | ○ | ○ | ○ | ○ |
| Creative | ○ | ○ | ○ | ○ | ○ |

**Ratings** ☆ ☆ ☆ ☆ ☆

# Strain

Grower

Acquired

Date

$

Indica      Hybrid      Sativa

☐ Flower     ☐ Edible     ☐ Concentrate

## Symptoms Relieved

## Notes

Sweet

Fruity      Floral

Sour      Spicy

Earthy      Herbal

Woodsy

| **Effects** | **Strength** | | | | |
|---|---|---|---|---|---|
| Peaceful | ○ | ○ | ○ | ○ | ○ |
| Sleepy | ○ | ○ | ○ | ○ | ○ |
| Pain Relief | ○ | ○ | ○ | ○ | ○ |
| Hungry | ○ | ○ | ○ | ○ | ○ |
| Uplifted | ○ | ○ | ○ | ○ | ○ |
| Creative | ○ | ○ | ○ | ○ | ○ |

**Ratings** ☆ ☆ ☆ ☆ ☆

# Strain

Grower

Date

Acquired

$

| Indica | Hybrid | Sativa |

☐ Flower  ☐ Edible  ☐ Concentrate

## Symptoms Relieved

## Notes

Sweet
Fruity
Floral
Sour
Spicy
Earthy
Herbal
Woodsy

| **Effects** | **Strength** |

Peaceful ○ ○ ○ ○ ○

Sleepy ○ ○ ○ ○ ○

Pain Relief ○ ○ ○ ○ ○

Hungry ○ ○ ○ ○ ○

Uplifted ○ ○ ○ ○ ○

Creative ○ ○ ○ ○ ○

**Ratings** ☆ ☆ ☆ ☆ ☆

# Strain

Grower

Date

Acquired

$

|  Indica | Hybrid | Sativa |

☐ Flower   ☐ Edible   ☐ Concentrate

## Symptoms Relieved

Sweet

Fruity

Floral

Sour

Spicy

Earthy

Herbal

Woodsy

## Notes

| Effects | Strength |
| --- | --- |
| Peaceful | ○ ○ ○ ○ ○ |
| Sleepy | ○ ○ ○ ○ ○ |
| Pain Relief | ○ ○ ○ ○ ○ |
| Hungry | ○ ○ ○ ○ ○ |
| Uplifted | ○ ○ ○ ○ ○ |
| Creative | ○ ○ ○ ○ ○ |

**Ratings** ☆ ☆ ☆ ☆ ☆

# Strain

Grower

Date

Acquired

$

| Indica | Hybrid | Sativa |
| --- | --- | --- |

☐ Flower  ☐ Edible  ☐ Concentrate

## Symptoms Relieved



## Notes

| Effects | Strength |
| --- | --- |
| Peaceful | ○ ○ ○ ○ ○ |
| Sleepy | ○ ○ ○ ○ ○ |
| Pain Relief | ○ ○ ○ ○ ○ |
| Hungry | ○ ○ ○ ○ ○ |
| Uplifted | ○ ○ ○ ○ ○ |
| Creative | ○ ○ ○ ○ ○ |

**Ratings** ☆ ☆ ☆ ☆ ☆

# Strain

Grower

Date

Acquired

$

| Indica | Hybrid | Sativa |

☐ Flower    ☐ Edible    ☐ Concentrate

## Symptoms Relieved

Sweet
Fruity
Floral
Sour
Spicy
Earthy
Herbal
Woodsy

## Notes

| **Effects** | **Strength** |

Peaceful ○ ○ ○ ○ ○

Sleepy ○ ○ ○ ○ ○

Pain Relief ○ ○ ○ ○ ○

Hungry ○ ○ ○ ○ ○

Uplifted ○ ○ ○ ○ ○

Creative ○ ○ ○ ○ ○

**Ratings** ☆ ☆ ☆ ☆ ☆

# Strain

Grower

Date

Acquired

$

| Indica | Hybrid | Sativa |

☐ Flower    ☐ Edible    ☐ Concentrate

## Symptoms Relieved

Sweet
Fruity
Floral
Sour
Spicy
Earthy
Herbal
Woodsy

## Notes

| **Effects** | **Strength** |

Peaceful   ○ ○ ○ ○ ○

Sleepy   ○ ○ ○ ○ ○

Pain Relief   ○ ○ ○ ○ ○

Hungry   ○ ○ ○ ○ ○

Uplifted   ○ ○ ○ ○ ○

Creative   ○ ○ ○ ○ ○

**Ratings**   ☆ ☆ ☆ ☆ ☆

# Strain

Grower

Date

Acquired

$

| Indica | Hybrid | Sativa |

☐ Flower   ☐ Edible   ☐ Concentrate

## Symptoms Relieved

Sweet

Fruity

Floral

Sour

Spicy

Earthy

Herbal

Woodsy

## Notes

| Effects | Strength |
| --- | --- |
| Peaceful | ○ ○ ○ ○ ○ |
| Sleepy | ○ ○ ○ ○ ○ |
| Pain Relief | ○ ○ ○ ○ ○ |
| Hungry | ○ ○ ○ ○ ○ |
| Uplifted | ○ ○ ○ ○ ○ |
| Creative | ○ ○ ○ ○ ○ |

**Ratings** ☆ ☆ ☆ ☆ ☆

# Strain

Grower ___________________________  Date _______________

Acquired _________________________  $ _______________

| Indica | Hybrid | Sativa |
| --- | --- | --- |

☐ Flower   ☐ Edible   ☐ Concentrate

## Symptoms Relieved

Sweet
Fruity
Floral
Sour
Spicy
Earthy
Herbal
Woodsy

## Notes

| Effects | Strength | | | | |
| --- | --- | --- | --- | --- | --- |
| Peaceful | ○ | ○ | ○ | ○ | ○ |
| Sleepy | ○ | ○ | ○ | ○ | ○ |
| Pain Relief | ○ | ○ | ○ | ○ | ○ |
| Hungry | ○ | ○ | ○ | ○ | ○ |
| Uplifted | ○ | ○ | ○ | ○ | ○ |
| Creative | ○ | ○ | ○ | ○ | ○ |

**Ratings** ☆ ☆ ☆ ☆ ☆

# Strain

Grower

Date

Acquired

$

| Indica | Hybrid | Sativa |

☐ Flower  ☐ Edible  ☐ Concentrate

## Symptoms Relieved

Sweet

Fruity

Floral

Sour

Spicy

Earthy

Herbal

Woodsy

## Notes

| Effects | Strength |

Peaceful ○ ○ ○ ○ ○

Sleepy ○ ○ ○ ○ ○

Pain Relief ○ ○ ○ ○ ○

Hungry ○ ○ ○ ○ ○

Uplifted ○ ○ ○ ○ ○

Creative ○ ○ ○ ○ ○

**Ratings** ☆ ☆ ☆ ☆ ☆

# Strain

Grower

Acquired

Date

$

| Indica | Hybrid | Sativa |

☐ Flower  ☐ Edible  ☐ Concentrate

## Symptoms Relieved

## Notes

Sweet

Fruity

Floral

Sour

Spicy

Earthy

Herbal

Woodsy

| Effects | Strength |
| --- | --- |
| Peaceful | ○ ○ ○ ○ ○ |
| Sleepy | ○ ○ ○ ○ ○ |
| Pain Relief | ○ ○ ○ ○ ○ |
| Hungry | ○ ○ ○ ○ ○ |
| Uplifted | ○ ○ ○ ○ ○ |
| Creative | ○ ○ ○ ○ ○ |

**Ratings** ☆ ☆ ☆ ☆ ☆

# Strain

Grower

Date

Acquired

$

|  Indica | Hybrid | Sativa |

☐ Flower   ☐ Edible   ☐ Concentrate

## Symptoms Relieved

Sweet

Fruity

Floral

Sour

Spicy

Earthy

Herbal

Woodsy

## Notes

| **Effects** | **Strength** |

Peaceful   ○ ○ ○ ○ ○

Sleepy   ○ ○ ○ ○ ○

Pain Relief   ○ ○ ○ ○ ○

Hungry   ○ ○ ○ ○ ○

Uplifted   ○ ○ ○ ○ ○

Creative   ○ ○ ○ ○ ○

**Ratings**   ☆ ☆ ☆ ☆ ☆

# Strain

Grower

Date

Acquired

$

| Indica | Hybrid | Sativa |

☐ Flower  ☐ Edible  ☐ Concentrate

## Symptoms Relieved

Sweet

Fruity

Floral

Sour

Spicy

Earthy

Herbal

Woodsy

## Notes

| **Effects** | **Strength** |

Peaceful ○ ○ ○ ○ ○

Sleepy ○ ○ ○ ○ ○

Pain Relief ○ ○ ○ ○ ○

Hungry ○ ○ ○ ○ ○

Uplifted ○ ○ ○ ○ ○

Creative ○ ○ ○ ○ ○

**Ratings** ☆ ☆ ☆ ☆ ☆

# Strain

Grower

Date

Acquired

$

|  |  |  |
|---|---|---|
| Indica | Hybrid | Sativa |

☐ Flower    ☐ Edible    ☐ Concentrate

## Symptoms Relieved



## Notes

| Effects | Strength | | | | |
|---|---|---|---|---|---|
| Peaceful | ○ | ○ | ○ | ○ | ○ |
| Sleepy | ○ | ○ | ○ | ○ | ○ |
| Pain Relief | ○ | ○ | ○ | ○ | ○ |
| Hungry | ○ | ○ | ○ | ○ | ○ |
| Uplifted | ○ | ○ | ○ | ○ | ○ |
| Creative | ○ | ○ | ○ | ○ | ○ |

**Ratings** ☆ ☆ ☆ ☆ ☆

# Strain

Grower

Date

Acquired

$

| Indica | Hybrid | Sativa |

☐ Flower  ☐ Edible  ☐ Concentrate

## Symptoms Relieved

## Notes



| Effects | Strength |
| --- | --- |
| Peaceful | ○ ○ ○ ○ ○ |
| Sleepy | ○ ○ ○ ○ ○ |
| Pain Relief | ○ ○ ○ ○ ○ |
| Hungry | ○ ○ ○ ○ ○ |
| Uplifted | ○ ○ ○ ○ ○ |
| Creative | ○ ○ ○ ○ ○ |

**Ratings** ☆ ☆ ☆ ☆ ☆

# Strain

Grower

Acquired

Date

$

| Indica | Hybrid | Sativa |

☐ Flower  ☐ Edible  ☐ Concentrate

## Symptoms Relieved

Sweet
Fruity
Floral
Sour
Spicy
Earthy
Herbal
Woodsy

## Notes

| Effects | Strength |
| --- | --- |
| Peaceful | ○ ○ ○ ○ ○ |
| Sleepy | ○ ○ ○ ○ ○ |
| Pain Relief | ○ ○ ○ ○ ○ |
| Hungry | ○ ○ ○ ○ ○ |
| Uplifted | ○ ○ ○ ○ ○ |
| Creative | ○ ○ ○ ○ ○ |

**Ratings** ☆ ☆ ☆ ☆ ☆

# Strain

Grower

Date

Acquired

$

|  |  |  |
|---|---|---|
| Indica | Hybrid | Sativa |

☐ Flower          ☐ Edible          ☐ Concentrate

## Symptoms Relieved

Sweet
Fruity
Floral
Sour
Spicy
Earthy
Herbal
Woodsy

## Notes

| **Effects** | **Strength** | | | | |
|---|---|---|---|---|---|
| Peaceful | ○ | ○ | ○ | ○ | ○ |
| Sleepy | ○ | ○ | ○ | ○ | ○ |
| Pain Relief | ○ | ○ | ○ | ○ | ○ |
| Hungry | ○ | ○ | ○ | ○ | ○ |
| Uplifted | ○ | ○ | ○ | ○ | ○ |
| Creative | ○ | ○ | ○ | ○ | ○ |

**Ratings** ☆ ☆ ☆ ☆ ☆

# Strain

Grower

Date

Acquired

$

| Indica | Hybrid | Sativa |

☐ Flower    ☐ Edible    ☐ Concentrate

## Symptoms Relieved

Sweet

Fruity    Floral

Sour    Spicy

Earthy    Herbal

Woodsy

## Notes

| Effects | Strength |
| --- | --- |
| Peaceful | ○ ○ ○ ○ ○ |
| Sleepy | ○ ○ ○ ○ ○ |
| Pain Relief | ○ ○ ○ ○ ○ |
| Hungry | ○ ○ ○ ○ ○ |
| Uplifted | ○ ○ ○ ○ ○ |
| Creative | ○ ○ ○ ○ ○ |

**Ratings** ☆ ☆ ☆ ☆ ☆

# Strain

Grower

Acquired

Date

$

|  |  |  |
|---|---|---|
| Indica | Hybrid | Sativa |

☐ Flower     ☐ Edible     ☐ Concentrate

## Symptoms Relieved

## Notes

Sweet

Fruity

Floral

Sour

Spicy

Earthy

Herbal

Woodsy

| Effects | Strength |
|---|---|
| Peaceful | ○ ○ ○ ○ ○ |
| Sleepy | ○ ○ ○ ○ ○ |
| Pain Relief | ○ ○ ○ ○ ○ |
| Hungry | ○ ○ ○ ○ ○ |
| Uplifted | ○ ○ ○ ○ ○ |
| Creative | ○ ○ ○ ○ ○ |

**Ratings** ☆ ☆ ☆ ☆ ☆

# Strain

Grower

Date

Acquired

$

| Indica | Hybrid | Sativa |

☐ Flower ☐ Edible ☐ Concentrate

## Symptoms Relieved

Sweet

Fruity

Floral

Sour

Spicy

Earthy

Herbal

Woodsy

## Notes

| Effects | Strength |
| --- | --- |
| Peaceful | ○ ○ ○ ○ ○ |
| Sleepy | ○ ○ ○ ○ ○ |
| Pain Relief | ○ ○ ○ ○ ○ |
| Hungry | ○ ○ ○ ○ ○ |
| Uplifted | ○ ○ ○ ○ ○ |
| Creative | ○ ○ ○ ○ ○ |

**Ratings** ☆ ☆ ☆ ☆ ☆

# Strain

Grower

Date

Acquired

$

| Indica | Hybrid | Sativa |

☐ Flower    ☐ Edible    ☐ Concentrate

## Symptoms Relieved

## Notes

Sweet
Fruity
Floral
Sour
Spicy
Earthy
Herbal
Woodsy

| Effects | Strength |
| --- | --- |
| Peaceful | ○ ○ ○ ○ ○ |
| Sleepy | ○ ○ ○ ○ ○ |
| Pain Relief | ○ ○ ○ ○ ○ |
| Hungry | ○ ○ ○ ○ ○ |
| Uplifted | ○ ○ ○ ○ ○ |
| Creative | ○ ○ ○ ○ ○ |

**Ratings** ☆ ☆ ☆ ☆ ☆

# Strain

Grower

Date

Acquired

$

| Indica | Hybrid | Sativa |

☐ Flower   ☐ Edible   ☐ Concentrate

## Symptoms Relieved

## Notes



| Effects | Strength |
|---|---|
| Peaceful | ◯ ◯ ◯ ◯ ◯ |
| Sleepy | ◯ ◯ ◯ ◯ ◯ |
| Pain Relief | ◯ ◯ ◯ ◯ ◯ |
| Hungry | ◯ ◯ ◯ ◯ ◯ |
| Uplifted | ◯ ◯ ◯ ◯ ◯ |
| Creative | ◯ ◯ ◯ ◯ ◯ |

**Ratings** ☆ ☆ ☆ ☆ ☆

# Strain

Grower

Date

Acquired

$

|  Indica | Hybrid | Sativa |

☐ Flower  ☐ Edible  ☐ Concentrate

## Symptoms Relieved

## Notes

Sweet

Fruity

Floral

Sour

Spicy

Earthy

Herbal

Woodsy

| **Effects** | **Strength** |
| Peaceful | ○ ○ ○ ○ ○ |
| Sleepy | ○ ○ ○ ○ ○ |
| Pain Relief | ○ ○ ○ ○ ○ |
| Hungry | ○ ○ ○ ○ ○ |
| Uplifted | ○ ○ ○ ○ ○ |
| Creative | ○ ○ ○ ○ ○ |

**Ratings** ☆ ☆ ☆ ☆ ☆

# Strain

Grower

Date

Acquired

$

| Indica | Hybrid | Sativa |

☐ Flower  ☐ Edible  ☐ Concentrate

## Symptoms Relieved

Sweet

Fruity

Floral

Sour

Spicy

Earthy

Herbal

Woodsy

## Notes

| Effects | Strength |
| --- | --- |
| Peaceful | ○ ○ ○ ○ ○ |
| Sleepy | ○ ○ ○ ○ ○ |
| Pain Relief | ○ ○ ○ ○ ○ |
| Hungry | ○ ○ ○ ○ ○ |
| Uplifted | ○ ○ ○ ○ ○ |
| Creative | ○ ○ ○ ○ ○ |

**Ratings** ☆ ☆ ☆ ☆ ☆

# Strain

Grower

Date

Acquired

$

| Indica | Hybrid | Sativa |

☐ Flower  ☐ Edible  ☐ Concentrate

## Symptoms Relieved

Sweet

Fruity

Floral

Sour

Spicy

Earthy

Herbal

Woodsy

## Notes

| **Effects** | **Strength** |

Peaceful  ○ ○ ○ ○ ○

Sleepy  ○ ○ ○ ○ ○

Pain Relief  ○ ○ ○ ○ ○

Hungry  ○ ○ ○ ○ ○

Uplifted  ○ ○ ○ ○ ○

Creative  ○ ○ ○ ○ ○

**Ratings**  ☆ ☆ ☆ ☆ ☆

# Strain

Grower

Acquired

Date

$

| Indica | Hybrid | Sativa |

☐ Flower  ☐ Edible  ☐ Concentrate

## Symptoms Relieved

Sweet

Fruity

Floral

Sour

Spicy

Earthy

Herbal

Woodsy

## Notes

| Effects | Strength |

Peaceful ○ ○ ○ ○ ○

Sleepy ○ ○ ○ ○ ○

Pain Relief ○ ○ ○ ○ ○

Hungry ○ ○ ○ ○ ○

Uplifted ○ ○ ○ ○ ○

Creative ○ ○ ○ ○ ○

**Ratings** ☆ ☆ ☆ ☆ ☆

# Strain

Grower

Acquired

Date

$

| Indica | Hybrid | Sativa |
| --- | --- | --- |

☐ Flower     ☐ Edible     ☐ Concentrate

## Symptoms Relieved

Sweet

Fruity

Floral

Sour

Spicy

Earthy

Herbal

Woodsy

## Notes

| Effects | Strength | | | | |
| --- | --- | --- | --- | --- | --- |
| Peaceful | ○ | ○ | ○ | ○ | ○ |
| Sleepy | ○ | ○ | ○ | ○ | ○ |
| Pain Relief | ○ | ○ | ○ | ○ | ○ |
| Hungry | ○ | ○ | ○ | ○ | ○ |
| Uplifted | ○ | ○ | ○ | ○ | ○ |
| Creative | ○ | ○ | ○ | ○ | ○ |

**Ratings** ☆ ☆ ☆ ☆ ☆

# Strain

Grower

Date

Acquired

$

| Indica | Hybrid | Sativa |

☐ Flower    ☐ Edible    ☐ Concentrate

## Symptoms Relieved



## Notes

| Effects | Strength | | | | |
| --- | --- | --- | --- | --- | --- |
| Peaceful | ○ | ○ | ○ | ○ | ○ |
| Sleepy | ○ | ○ | ○ | ○ | ○ |
| Pain Relief | ○ | ○ | ○ | ○ | ○ |
| Hungry | ○ | ○ | ○ | ○ | ○ |
| Uplifted | ○ | ○ | ○ | ○ | ○ |
| Creative | ○ | ○ | ○ | ○ | ○ |

**Ratings** ☆ ☆ ☆ ☆ ☆

# Strain

Grower

Date

Acquired

$

| Indica | Hybrid | Sativa |

☐ Flower   ☐ Edible   ☐ Concentrate

## Symptoms Relieved

## Notes

**Sweet**

**Fruity**

**Floral**

**Sour**

**Spicy**

**Earthy**

**Herbal**

**Woodsy**

| **Effects** | **Strength** |
| --- | --- |
| Peaceful | ○ ○ ○ ○ ○ |
| Sleepy | ○ ○ ○ ○ ○ |
| Pain Relief | ○ ○ ○ ○ ○ |
| Hungry | ○ ○ ○ ○ ○ |
| Uplifted | ○ ○ ○ ○ ○ |
| Creative | ○ ○ ○ ○ ○ |

**Ratings** ☆ ☆ ☆ ☆ ☆

# Strain

Grower

Acquired

Date

$

|  Indica | Hybrid | Sativa |
| --- | --- | --- |

☐ Flower    ☐ Edible    ☐ Concentrate

## Symptoms Relieved

Sweet
Fruity
Floral
Sour
Spicy
Earthy
Herbal
Woodsy

## Notes

| Effects | Strength | | | | |
| --- | --- | --- | --- | --- | --- |
| Peaceful | ◯ | ◯ | ◯ | ◯ | ◯ |
| Sleepy | ◯ | ◯ | ◯ | ◯ | ◯ |
| Pain Relief | ◯ | ◯ | ◯ | ◯ | ◯ |
| Hungry | ◯ | ◯ | ◯ | ◯ | ◯ |
| Uplifted | ◯ | ◯ | ◯ | ◯ | ◯ |
| Creative | ◯ | ◯ | ◯ | ◯ | ◯ |

**Ratings** ☆ ☆ ☆ ☆ ☆

# Strain

Grower

Date

Acquired

$

| Indica | Hybrid | Sativa |

☐ Flower     ☐ Edible     ☐ Concentrate

## Symptoms Relieved

## Notes

**Sweet**

**Fruity**

**Floral**

**Sour**

**Spicy**

**Earthy**

**Herbal**

**Woodsy**

| **Effects** | **Strength** |
|---|---|
| Peaceful | ◯ ◯ ◯ ◯ ◯ |
| Sleepy | ◯ ◯ ◯ ◯ ◯ |
| Pain Relief | ◯ ◯ ◯ ◯ ◯ |
| Hungry | ◯ ◯ ◯ ◯ ◯ |
| Uplifted | ◯ ◯ ◯ ◯ ◯ |
| Creative | ◯ ◯ ◯ ◯ ◯ |

**Ratings** ☆ ☆ ☆ ☆ ☆

# Strain

Grower

Date

Acquired

$

| Indica | Hybrid | Sativa |

☐ Flower  ☐ Edible  ☐ Concentrate

## Symptoms Relieved



## Notes

| Effects | Strength |
| --- | --- |
| Peaceful | ◯ ◯ ◯ ◯ ◯ |
| Sleepy | ◯ ◯ ◯ ◯ ◯ |
| Pain Relief | ◯ ◯ ◯ ◯ ◯ |
| Hungry | ◯ ◯ ◯ ◯ ◯ |
| Uplifted | ◯ ◯ ◯ ◯ ◯ |
| Creative | ◯ ◯ ◯ ◯ ◯ |

**Ratings** ☆ ☆ ☆ ☆ ☆

# Strain

Grower

Date

Acquired

$

| Indica | Hybrid | Sativa |

☐ Flower    ☐ Edible    ☐ Concentrate

## Symptoms Relieved



## Notes

| Effects | Strength |
| --- | --- |
| Peaceful | ○ ○ ○ ○ ○ |
| Sleepy | ○ ○ ○ ○ ○ |
| Pain Relief | ○ ○ ○ ○ ○ |
| Hungry | ○ ○ ○ ○ ○ |
| Uplifted | ○ ○ ○ ○ ○ |
| Creative | ○ ○ ○ ○ ○ |

**Ratings** ☆ ☆ ☆ ☆ ☆

# Strain

Grower

Date

Acquired

$

|  Indica | Hybrid | Sativa |
| --- | --- | --- |

☐ Flower    ☐ Edible    ☐ Concentrate

## Symptoms Relieved

Sweet
Fruity
Floral
Sour
Spicy
Earthy
Herbal
Woodsy

## Notes

| Effects | Strength |
| --- | --- |
| Peaceful | ○ ○ ○ ○ ○ |
| Sleepy | ○ ○ ○ ○ ○ |
| Pain Relief | ○ ○ ○ ○ ○ |
| Hungry | ○ ○ ○ ○ ○ |
| Uplifted | ○ ○ ○ ○ ○ |
| Creative | ○ ○ ○ ○ ○ |

**Ratings** ☆ ☆ ☆ ☆ ☆

# Strain

Grower

Date

Acquired

$

| Indica | Hybrid | Sativa |

☐ Flower  ☐ Edible  ☐ Concentrate

## Symptoms Relieved

Sweet
Fruity
Floral
Sour
Spicy
Earthy
Herbal
Woodsy

## Notes

| Effects | Strength |
| --- | --- |
| Peaceful | ◯ ◯ ◯ ◯ ◯ |
| Sleepy | ◯ ◯ ◯ ◯ ◯ |
| Pain Relief | ◯ ◯ ◯ ◯ ◯ |
| Hungry | ◯ ◯ ◯ ◯ ◯ |
| Uplifted | ◯ ◯ ◯ ◯ ◯ |
| Creative | ◯ ◯ ◯ ◯ ◯ |

**Ratings** ☆ ☆ ☆ ☆ ☆

# Strain

Grower

Date

Acquired

$

| Indica | Hybrid | Sativa |

☐ Flower  ☐ Edible  ☐ Concentrate

## Symptoms Relieved

Sweet

Fruity

Floral

Sour

Spicy

Earthy

Herbal

Woodsy

## Notes

| Effects | Strength | | | | |
| --- | --- | --- | --- | --- | --- |
| Peaceful | ○ | ○ | ○ | ○ | ○ |
| Sleepy | ○ | ○ | ○ | ○ | ○ |
| Pain Relief | ○ | ○ | ○ | ○ | ○ |
| Hungry | ○ | ○ | ○ | ○ | ○ |
| Uplifted | ○ | ○ | ○ | ○ | ○ |
| Creative | ○ | ○ | ○ | ○ | ○ |

**Ratings** ☆ ☆ ☆ ☆ ☆

# Strain

Grower

Date

Acquired

$

| Indica | Hybrid | Sativa |

☐ Flower     ☐ Edible     ☐ Concentrate

## Symptoms Relieved

Sweet

Fruity

Floral

Sour

Spicy

Earthy

Herbal

Woodsy

## Notes

| Effects | Strength |
| --- | --- |
| Peaceful | ○ ○ ○ ○ ○ |
| Sleepy | ○ ○ ○ ○ ○ |
| Pain Relief | ○ ○ ○ ○ ○ |
| Hungry | ○ ○ ○ ○ ○ |
| Uplifted | ○ ○ ○ ○ ○ |
| Creative | ○ ○ ○ ○ ○ |

**Ratings** ☆ ☆ ☆ ☆ ☆

# Strain

Grower

Date

Acquired

$

| Indica | Hybrid | Sativa |

☐ Flower ☐ Edible ☐ Concentrate

## Symptoms Relieved

## Notes

Sweet

Fruity

Floral

Sour

Spicy

Earthy

Herbal

Woodsy

| Effects | Strength |

Peaceful ○ ○ ○ ○ ○

Sleepy ○ ○ ○ ○ ○

Pain Relief ○ ○ ○ ○ ○

Hungry ○ ○ ○ ○ ○

Uplifted ○ ○ ○ ○ ○

Creative ○ ○ ○ ○ ○

**Ratings** ☆ ☆ ☆ ☆ ☆

# Strain

Grower

Date

Acquired

$

| Indica | Hybrid | Sativa |

☐ Flower   ☐ Edible   ☐ Concentrate

## Symptoms Relieved

## Notes

Sweet

Fruity

Floral

Sour

Spicy

Earthy

Herbal

Woodsy

| Effects | Strength |
| --- | --- |
| Peaceful | ○ ○ ○ ○ ○ |
| Sleepy | ○ ○ ○ ○ ○ |
| Pain Relief | ○ ○ ○ ○ ○ |
| Hungry | ○ ○ ○ ○ ○ |
| Uplifted | ○ ○ ○ ○ ○ |
| Creative | ○ ○ ○ ○ ○ |

**Ratings** ☆ ☆ ☆ ☆ ☆

# Strain

Grower

Date

Acquired

$

| Indica | Hybrid | Sativa |

☐ Flower  ☐ Edible  ☐ Concentrate

## Symptoms Relieved

Sweet

Fruity

Floral

Sour

Spicy

Earthy

Herbal

Woodsy

## Notes

| Effects | Strength |
| --- | --- |
| Peaceful | ○ ○ ○ ○ ○ |
| Sleepy | ○ ○ ○ ○ ○ |
| Pain Relief | ○ ○ ○ ○ ○ |
| Hungry | ○ ○ ○ ○ ○ |
| Uplifted | ○ ○ ○ ○ ○ |
| Creative | ○ ○ ○ ○ ○ |

**Ratings** ☆ ☆ ☆ ☆ ☆

# Strain

Grower

Acquired

Date

$

| Indica | Hybrid | Sativa |

☐ Flower ☐ Edible ☐ Concentrate

## Symptoms Relieved

Sweet

Fruity

Floral

Sour

Spicy

Earthy

Herbal

Woodsy

## Notes

| **Effects** | **Strength** |
|---|---|
| Peaceful | ◯ ◯ ◯ ◯ ◯ |
| Sleepy | ◯ ◯ ◯ ◯ ◯ |
| Pain Relief | ◯ ◯ ◯ ◯ ◯ |
| Hungry | ◯ ◯ ◯ ◯ ◯ |
| Uplifted | ◯ ◯ ◯ ◯ ◯ |
| Creative | ◯ ◯ ◯ ◯ ◯ |

**Ratings** ☆ ☆ ☆ ☆ ☆

# Strain

Grower

Date

Acquired

$

|  |  |  |
|---|---|---|
| Indica | Hybrid | Sativa |

☐ Flower    ☐ Edible    ☐ Concentrate

## Symptoms Relieved



## Notes

| Effects | Strength | | | | |
|---|---|---|---|---|---|
| Peaceful | ○ | ○ | ○ | ○ | ○ |
| Sleepy | ○ | ○ | ○ | ○ | ○ |
| Pain Relief | ○ | ○ | ○ | ○ | ○ |
| Hungry | ○ | ○ | ○ | ○ | ○ |
| Uplifted | ○ | ○ | ○ | ○ | ○ |
| Creative | ○ | ○ | ○ | ○ | ○ |

**Ratings**  ☆ ☆ ☆ ☆ ☆

# Strain

Grower

Date

Acquired

$

| Indica | Hybrid | Sativa |

☐ Flower   ☐ Edible   ☐ Concentrate

## Symptoms Relieved

Sweet

Fruity

Floral

Sour

Spicy

Earthy

Herbal

Woodsy

## Notes

| **Effects** | **Strength** |

Peaceful ○ ○ ○ ○ ○

Sleepy ○ ○ ○ ○ ○

Pain Relief ○ ○ ○ ○ ○

Hungry ○ ○ ○ ○ ○

Uplifted ○ ○ ○ ○ ○

Creative ○ ○ ○ ○ ○

**Ratings** ☆ ☆ ☆ ☆ ☆

# Strain

Grower

Date

Acquired

$

| Indica | Hybrid | Sativa |

☐ Flower ☐ Edible ☐ Concentrate

## Symptoms Relieved



## Notes

| **Effects** | **Strength** | | | | |
| --- | --- | --- | --- | --- | --- |
| Peaceful | ◯ | ◯ | ◯ | ◯ | ◯ |
| Sleepy | ◯ | ◯ | ◯ | ◯ | ◯ |
| Pain Relief | ◯ | ◯ | ◯ | ◯ | ◯ |
| Hungry | ◯ | ◯ | ◯ | ◯ | ◯ |
| Uplifted | ◯ | ◯ | ◯ | ◯ | ◯ |
| Creative | ◯ | ◯ | ◯ | ◯ | ◯ |

**Ratings** ☆ ☆ ☆ ☆ ☆

# Strain

Grower

Date

Acquired

$

|  Indica | Hybrid | Sativa |

☐ Flower   ☐ Edible   ☐ Concentrate

## Symptoms Relieved

Sweet
Fruity
Floral
Sour
Spicy
Earthy
Herbal
Woodsy

## Notes

| Effects | Strength |
| --- | --- |
| Peaceful | ○ ○ ○ ○ ○ |
| Sleepy | ○ ○ ○ ○ ○ |
| Pain Relief | ○ ○ ○ ○ ○ |
| Hungry | ○ ○ ○ ○ ○ |
| Uplifted | ○ ○ ○ ○ ○ |
| Creative | ○ ○ ○ ○ ○ |

**Ratings** ☆ ☆ ☆ ☆ ☆

# Strain

Grower

Date

Acquired

$

|  |  |  |
|---|---|---|
| Indica | Hybrid | Sativa |

☐ Flower   ☐ Edible   ☐ Concentrate

## Symptoms Relieved

Sweet

Fruity

Floral

Sour

Spicy

Earthy

Herbal

Woodsy

## Notes

| Effects | Strength |
|---|---|
| Peaceful | ○ ○ ○ ○ ○ |
| Sleepy | ○ ○ ○ ○ ○ |
| Pain Relief | ○ ○ ○ ○ ○ |
| Hungry | ○ ○ ○ ○ ○ |
| Uplifted | ○ ○ ○ ○ ○ |
| Creative | ○ ○ ○ ○ ○ |

**Ratings** ☆ ☆ ☆ ☆ ☆

# Strain

Grower

Date

Acquired

$

| Indica | Hybrid | Sativa |

☐ Flower   ☐ Edible   ☐ Concentrate

## Symptoms Relieved

## Notes

**Effects**     **Strength**

Peaceful   ○ ○ ○ ○ ○

Sleepy   ○ ○ ○ ○ ○

Pain Relief   ○ ○ ○ ○ ○

Hungry   ○ ○ ○ ○ ○

Uplifted   ○ ○ ○ ○ ○

Creative   ○ ○ ○ ○ ○

**Ratings** ☆ ☆ ☆ ☆ ☆

Sweet · Floral · Spicy · Herbal · Woodsy · Earthy · Sour · Fruity

# Strain

Grower

Date

Acquired

$

| Indica | Hybrid | Sativa |

☐ Flower   ☐ Edible   ☐ Concentrate

## Symptoms Relieved

## Notes

Sweet

Fruity

Floral

Sour

Spicy

Earthy

Herbal

Woodsy

| **Effects** | **Strength** | | | | |
| --- | --- | --- | --- | --- | --- |
| Peaceful | ○ | ○ | ○ | ○ | ○ |
| Sleepy | ○ | ○ | ○ | ○ | ○ |
| Pain Relief | ○ | ○ | ○ | ○ | ○ |
| Hungry | ○ | ○ | ○ | ○ | ○ |
| Uplifted | ○ | ○ | ○ | ○ | ○ |
| Creative | ○ | ○ | ○ | ○ | ○ |

**Ratings** ☆ ☆ ☆ ☆ ☆

# Strain

Grower

Date

Acquired

$

| Indica | Hybrid | Sativa |
| --- | --- | --- |

☐ Flower  ☐ Edible  ☐ Concentrate

## Symptoms Relieved

Sweet

Fruity

Floral

Sour

Spicy

Earthy

Herbal

Woodsy

## Notes

| Effects | Strength | | | | |
| --- | --- | --- | --- | --- | --- |
| Peaceful | ◯ | ◯ | ◯ | ◯ | ◯ |
| Sleepy | ◯ | ◯ | ◯ | ◯ | ◯ |
| Pain Relief | ◯ | ◯ | ◯ | ◯ | ◯ |
| Hungry | ◯ | ◯ | ◯ | ◯ | ◯ |
| Uplifted | ◯ | ◯ | ◯ | ◯ | ◯ |
| Creative | ◯ | ◯ | ◯ | ◯ | ◯ |

**Ratings** ☆ ☆ ☆ ☆ ☆

# Strain

Grower

Date

Acquired

$

| Indica | Hybrid | Sativa |
| --- | --- | --- |

☐ Flower  ☐ Edible  ☐ Concentrate

## Symptoms Relieved

## Notes

Sweet
Fruity
Floral
Sour
Spicy
Earthy
Herbal
Woodsy

| **Effects** | **Strength** |
| --- | --- |
| Peaceful | ○ ○ ○ ○ ○ |
| Sleepy | ○ ○ ○ ○ ○ |
| Pain Relief | ○ ○ ○ ○ ○ |
| Hungry | ○ ○ ○ ○ ○ |
| Uplifted | ○ ○ ○ ○ ○ |
| Creative | ○ ○ ○ ○ ○ |

**Ratings** ☆ ☆ ☆ ☆ ☆

# Strain

Grower

Date

Acquired

$

| Indica | Hybrid | Sativa |

☐ Flower ☐ Edible ☐ Concentrate

## Symptoms Relieved

Sweet
Fruity
Floral
Sour
Spicy
Earthy
Herbal
Woodsy

## Notes

| **Effects** | **Strength** |
| --- | --- |
| Peaceful | ○ ○ ○ ○ ○ |
| Sleepy | ○ ○ ○ ○ ○ |
| Pain Relief | ○ ○ ○ ○ ○ |
| Hungry | ○ ○ ○ ○ ○ |
| Uplifted | ○ ○ ○ ○ ○ |
| Creative | ○ ○ ○ ○ ○ |

**Ratings** ☆ ☆ ☆ ☆ ☆

# Strain

Grower

Date

Acquired

$

| Indica | Hybrid | Sativa |

☐ Flower  ☐ Edible  ☐ Concentrate

## Symptoms Relieved

## Notes

Sweet

Fruity

Floral

Sour

Spicy

Earthy

Herbal

Woodsy

| **Effects** | **Strength** |

Peaceful ○ ○ ○ ○ ○

Sleepy ○ ○ ○ ○ ○

Pain Relief ○ ○ ○ ○ ○

Hungry ○ ○ ○ ○ ○

Uplifted ○ ○ ○ ○ ○

Creative ○ ○ ○ ○ ○

**Ratings** ☆ ☆ ☆ ☆ ☆

# Strain

Grower

Date

Acquired

$

| Indica | Hybrid | Sativa |

☐ Flower    ☐ Edible    ☐ Concentrate

## Symptoms Relieved

## Notes

**Sweet**
**Fruity**
**Floral**
**Sour**
**Spicy**
**Earthy**
**Herbal**
**Woodsy**

| **Effects** | **Strength** |
|---|---|
| Peaceful | ○ ○ ○ ○ ○ |
| Sleepy | ○ ○ ○ ○ ○ |
| Pain Relief | ○ ○ ○ ○ ○ |
| Hungry | ○ ○ ○ ○ ○ |
| Uplifted | ○ ○ ○ ○ ○ |
| Creative | ○ ○ ○ ○ ○ |

**Ratings** ☆ ☆ ☆ ☆ ☆

# Strain

Grower ___________________  Date ___________________

Acquired ___________________  $ ___________________

| Indica | Hybrid | Sativa |
|---|---|---|

☐ Flower   ☐ Edible   ☐ Concentrate

## Symptoms Relieved

_______________________________

_______________________________

_______________________________

Sweet

Fruity

Floral

Sour

Spicy

Earthy

Herbal

Woodsy

## Notes

_______________________________

_______________________________

_______________________________

_______________________________

_______________________________

_______________________________

_______________________________

_______________________________

| Effects | Strength | | | | |
|---|---|---|---|---|---|
| Peaceful | ○ | ○ | ○ | ○ | ○ |
| Sleepy | ○ | ○ | ○ | ○ | ○ |
| Pain Relief | ○ | ○ | ○ | ○ | ○ |
| Hungry | ○ | ○ | ○ | ○ | ○ |
| Uplifted | ○ | ○ | ○ | ○ | ○ |
| Creative | ○ | ○ | ○ | ○ | ○ |

**Ratings**  ☆ ☆ ☆ ☆ ☆

# Strain

Grower

Date

Acquired

$

| Indica | Hybrid | Sativa |

☐ Flower  ☐ Edible  ☐ Concentrate

## Symptoms Relieved

## Notes

Sweet

Fruity

Floral

Sour

Spicy

Earthy

Herbal

Woodsy

| Effects | Strength |
| --- | --- |
| Peaceful | ○ ○ ○ ○ ○ |
| Sleepy | ○ ○ ○ ○ ○ |
| Pain Relief | ○ ○ ○ ○ ○ |
| Hungry | ○ ○ ○ ○ ○ |
| Uplifted | ○ ○ ○ ○ ○ |
| Creative | ○ ○ ○ ○ ○ |

**Ratings** ☆ ☆ ☆ ☆ ☆

# Strain

Grower

Date

Acquired

$

<table>
<tr><td>Indica</td><td>Hybrid</td><td>Sativa</td></tr>
</table>

☐ Flower    ☐ Edible    ☐ Concentrate

## Symptoms Relieved

Sweet

Fruity

Floral

Sour

Spicy

Earthy

Herbal

Woodsy

## Notes

| Effects | Strength | | | | |
|---|---|---|---|---|---|
| Peaceful | ○ | ○ | ○ | ○ | ○ |
| Sleepy | ○ | ○ | ○ | ○ | ○ |
| Pain Relief | ○ | ○ | ○ | ○ | ○ |
| Hungry | ○ | ○ | ○ | ○ | ○ |
| Uplifted | ○ | ○ | ○ | ○ | ○ |
| Creative | ○ | ○ | ○ | ○ | ○ |

**Ratings** ☆ ☆ ☆ ☆ ☆

# Strain

Grower _______________________  Date _______________________

Acquired _______________________  $ _______________________

| Indica | Hybrid | Sativa |

☐ Flower   ☐ Edible   ☐ Concentrate

## Symptoms Relieved

## Notes

Sweet
Fruity
Floral
Sour
Spicy
Earthy
Herbal
Woodsy

| Effects | Strength |
| --- | --- |
| Peaceful | ○ ○ ○ ○ ○ |
| Sleepy | ○ ○ ○ ○ ○ |
| Pain Relief | ○ ○ ○ ○ ○ |
| Hungry | ○ ○ ○ ○ ○ |
| Uplifted | ○ ○ ○ ○ ○ |
| Creative | ○ ○ ○ ○ ○ |

**Ratings** ☆ ☆ ☆ ☆ ☆

# Strain

Grower ______________________    Date ______________

Acquired ______________________    $ ______________

<table>
<tr><td>Indica</td><td>Hybrid</td><td>Sativa</td></tr>
</table>

☐ Flower    ☐ Edible    ☐ Concentrate

## Symptoms Relieved

_______________________________________

_______________________________________

_______________________________________

_______________________________________

Sweet · Fruity · Floral · Sour · Spicy · Earthy · Woodsy · Herbal

## Notes

_______________________________________

_______________________________________

_______________________________________

_______________________________________

_______________________________________

_______________________________________

_______________________________________

_______________________________________

| Effects | Strength | | | | |
|---|---|---|---|---|---|
| Peaceful | ○ | ○ | ○ | ○ | ○ |
| Sleepy | ○ | ○ | ○ | ○ | ○ |
| Pain Relief | ○ | ○ | ○ | ○ | ○ |
| Hungry | ○ | ○ | ○ | ○ | ○ |
| Uplifted | ○ | ○ | ○ | ○ | ○ |
| Creative | ○ | ○ | ○ | ○ | ○ |

**Ratings** ☆ ☆ ☆ ☆ ☆

# Strain

Grower

Date

Acquired

$

| Indica | Hybrid | Sativa |
| --- | --- | --- |

☐ Flower    ☐ Edible    ☐ Concentrate

## Symptoms Relieved



## Notes

| Effects | Strength | | | | |
| --- | --- | --- | --- | --- | --- |
| Peaceful | ◯ | ◯ | ◯ | ◯ | ◯ |
| Sleepy | ◯ | ◯ | ◯ | ◯ | ◯ |
| Pain Relief | ◯ | ◯ | ◯ | ◯ | ◯ |
| Hungry | ◯ | ◯ | ◯ | ◯ | ◯ |
| Uplifted | ◯ | ◯ | ◯ | ◯ | ◯ |
| Creative | ◯ | ◯ | ◯ | ◯ | ◯ |

**Ratings** ☆ ☆ ☆ ☆ ☆

# Strain

Grower ___________________________  Date ___________

Acquired _________________________  $ _____________

| Indica | Hybrid | Sativa |
| --- | --- | --- |

☐ Flower  ☐ Edible  ☐ Concentrate

## Symptoms Relieved

_______________________________________

_______________________________________

_______________________________________

_______________________________________



## Notes

_______________________________________

_______________________________________

_______________________________________

_______________________________________

_______________________________________

_______________________________________

_______________________________________

_______________________________________

| Effects | Strength | | | | |
| --- | --- | --- | --- | --- | --- |
| Peaceful | ○ | ○ | ○ | ○ | ○ |
| Sleepy | ○ | ○ | ○ | ○ | ○ |
| Pain Relief | ○ | ○ | ○ | ○ | ○ |
| Hungry | ○ | ○ | ○ | ○ | ○ |
| Uplifted | ○ | ○ | ○ | ○ | ○ |
| Creative | ○ | ○ | ○ | ○ | ○ |

**Ratings** ☆ ☆ ☆ ☆ ☆

# Strain

Grower

Date

Acquired

$

| Indica | Hybrid | Sativa |

☐ Flower   ☐ Edible   ☐ Concentrate

## Symptoms Relieved



## Notes

| Effects | Strength |
| --- | --- |
| Peaceful | ○ ○ ○ ○ ○ |
| Sleepy | ○ ○ ○ ○ ○ |
| Pain Relief | ○ ○ ○ ○ ○ |
| Hungry | ○ ○ ○ ○ ○ |
| Uplifted | ○ ○ ○ ○ ○ |
| Creative | ○ ○ ○ ○ ○ |

**Ratings** ☆ ☆ ☆ ☆ ☆

# Strain

Grower

Date

Acquired

$

| Indica | Hybrid | Sativa |

☐ Flower  ☐ Edible  ☐ Concentrate

## Symptoms Relieved

## Notes



| Effects | Strength |
| --- | --- |
| Peaceful | ○ ○ ○ ○ ○ |
| Sleepy | ○ ○ ○ ○ ○ |
| Pain Relief | ○ ○ ○ ○ ○ |
| Hungry | ○ ○ ○ ○ ○ |
| Uplifted | ○ ○ ○ ○ ○ |
| Creative | ○ ○ ○ ○ ○ |

**Ratings** ☆ ☆ ☆ ☆ ☆

# Strain

Grower

Date

Acquired

$

| Indica | Hybrid | Sativa |

☐ Flower　　☐ Edible　　☐ Concentrate

## Symptoms Relieved

## Notes



| Effects | Strength | | | | |
|---|---|---|---|---|---|
| Peaceful | ○ | ○ | ○ | ○ | ○ |
| Sleepy | ○ | ○ | ○ | ○ | ○ |
| Pain Relief | ○ | ○ | ○ | ○ | ○ |
| Hungry | ○ | ○ | ○ | ○ | ○ |
| Uplifted | ○ | ○ | ○ | ○ | ○ |
| Creative | ○ | ○ | ○ | ○ | ○ |

**Ratings** ☆ ☆ ☆ ☆ ☆

# Strain

Grower

Date

Acquired

$

| Indica | Hybrid | Sativa |

☐ Flower  ☐ Edible  ☐ Concentrate

## Symptoms Relieved



## Notes

| Effects | Strength |
| --- | --- |
| Peaceful | ○ ○ ○ ○ ○ |
| Sleepy | ○ ○ ○ ○ ○ |
| Pain Relief | ○ ○ ○ ○ ○ |
| Hungry | ○ ○ ○ ○ ○ |
| Uplifted | ○ ○ ○ ○ ○ |
| Creative | ○ ○ ○ ○ ○ |

**Ratings** ☆ ☆ ☆ ☆ ☆

# Strain

Grower

Acquired

Date

$

| Indica | Hybrid | Sativa |

☐ Flower  ☐ Edible  ☐ Concentrate

## Symptoms Relieved

## Notes

Sweet
Fruity
Floral
Sour
Spicy
Earthy
Herbal
Woodsy

| Effects | Strength |
| --- | --- |
| Peaceful | ○ ○ ○ ○ ○ |
| Sleepy | ○ ○ ○ ○ ○ |
| Pain Relief | ○ ○ ○ ○ ○ |
| Hungry | ○ ○ ○ ○ ○ |
| Uplifted | ○ ○ ○ ○ ○ |
| Creative | ○ ○ ○ ○ ○ |

**Ratings** ☆ ☆ ☆ ☆ ☆

# Strain

Grower

Date

Acquired

$

| Indica | Hybrid | Sativa |

☐ Flower   ☐ Edible   ☐ Concentrate

## Symptoms Relieved



## Notes

| Effects | Strength |
| --- | --- |
| Peaceful | ○ ○ ○ ○ ○ |
| Sleepy | ○ ○ ○ ○ ○ |
| Pain Relief | ○ ○ ○ ○ ○ |
| Hungry | ○ ○ ○ ○ ○ |
| Uplifted | ○ ○ ○ ○ ○ |
| Creative | ○ ○ ○ ○ ○ |

**Ratings** ☆ ☆ ☆ ☆ ☆

# Strain

Grower

Date

Acquired

$

| Indica | Hybrid | Sativa |
| --- | --- | --- |

☐ Flower  ☐ Edible  ☐ Concentrate

## Symptoms Relieved

Sweet

Fruity

Floral

Sour

Spicy

Earthy

Herbal

Woodsy

## Notes

| Effects | Strength |
| --- | --- |
| Peaceful | ○ ○ ○ ○ ○ |
| Sleepy | ○ ○ ○ ○ ○ |
| Pain Relief | ○ ○ ○ ○ ○ |
| Hungry | ○ ○ ○ ○ ○ |
| Uplifted | ○ ○ ○ ○ ○ |
| Creative | ○ ○ ○ ○ ○ |

**Ratings** ☆ ☆ ☆ ☆ ☆

# Strain

Grower

Date

Acquired

$

| Indica | Hybrid | Sativa |

☐ Flower   ☐ Edible   ☐ Concentrate

## Symptoms Relieved



## Notes

| Effects | Strength | | | | |
|---|---|---|---|---|---|
| Peaceful | ◯ | ◯ | ◯ | ◯ | ◯ |
| Sleepy | ◯ | ◯ | ◯ | ◯ | ◯ |
| Pain Relief | ◯ | ◯ | ◯ | ◯ | ◯ |
| Hungry | ◯ | ◯ | ◯ | ◯ | ◯ |
| Uplifted | ◯ | ◯ | ◯ | ◯ | ◯ |
| Creative | ◯ | ◯ | ◯ | ◯ | ◯ |

**Ratings** ☆ ☆ ☆ ☆ ☆

# Strain

Grower ___________________________  Date ___________________

Acquired _________________________  $ _____________________

| Indica | Hybrid | Sativa |

☐ Flower    ☐ Edible    ☐ Concentrate

## Symptoms Relieved

________________________________________________

________________________________________________

________________________________________________

________________________________________________

Sweet · Floral · Spicy · Herbal · Woodsy · Earthy · Sour · Fruity

## Notes

________________________________________________

________________________________________________

________________________________________________

________________________________________________

________________________________________________

________________________________________________

________________________________________________

________________________________________________

| Effects | Strength | | | | |
|---|---|---|---|---|---|
| Peaceful | ○ | ○ | ○ | ○ | ○ |
| Sleepy | ○ | ○ | ○ | ○ | ○ |
| Pain Relief | ○ | ○ | ○ | ○ | ○ |
| Hungry | ○ | ○ | ○ | ○ | ○ |
| Uplifted | ○ | ○ | ○ | ○ | ○ |
| Creative | ○ | ○ | ○ | ○ | ○ |

**Ratings** ☆ ☆ ☆ ☆ ☆

# Strain

Grower

Date

Acquired

$

| Indica | Hybrid | Sativa |

☐ Flower   ☐ Edible   ☐ Concentrate

## Symptoms Relieved

## Notes



| Effects | Strength |
| --- | --- |
| Peaceful | ○ ○ ○ ○ ○ |
| Sleepy | ○ ○ ○ ○ ○ |
| Pain Relief | ○ ○ ○ ○ ○ |
| Hungry | ○ ○ ○ ○ ○ |
| Uplifted | ○ ○ ○ ○ ○ |
| Creative | ○ ○ ○ ○ ○ |

**Ratings** ☆ ☆ ☆ ☆ ☆

# Strain

Grower

Date

Acquired

$

| Indica | Hybrid | Sativa |

☐ Flower  ☐ Edible  ☐ Concentrate

## Symptoms Relieved

Sweet
Fruity
Floral
Sour
Spicy
Earthy
Herbal
Woodsy

## Notes

| Effects | Strength | | | | |
| --- | --- | --- | --- | --- | --- |
| Peaceful | ○ | ○ | ○ | ○ | ○ |
| Sleepy | ○ | ○ | ○ | ○ | ○ |
| Pain Relief | ○ | ○ | ○ | ○ | ○ |
| Hungry | ○ | ○ | ○ | ○ | ○ |
| Uplifted | ○ | ○ | ○ | ○ | ○ |
| Creative | ○ | ○ | ○ | ○ | ○ |

**Ratings** ☆ ☆ ☆ ☆ ☆

# Strain

Grower

Date

Acquired

$

| Indica | Hybrid | Sativa |

☐ Flower    ☐ Edible    ☐ Concentrate

## Symptoms Relieved

Sweet

Fruity

Floral

Sour

Spicy

Earthy

Herbal

Woodsy

## Notes

| Effects | Strength |
| --- | --- |
| Peaceful | ○ ○ ○ ○ ○ |
| Sleepy | ○ ○ ○ ○ ○ |
| Pain Relief | ○ ○ ○ ○ ○ |
| Hungry | ○ ○ ○ ○ ○ |
| Uplifted | ○ ○ ○ ○ ○ |
| Creative | ○ ○ ○ ○ ○ |

**Ratings** ☆ ☆ ☆ ☆ ☆

# Strain

Grower

Date

Acquired

$

| Indica | Hybrid | Sativa |

☐ Flower   ☐ Edible   ☐ Concentrate

## Symptoms Relieved



## Notes

| Effects | Strength |
| --- | --- |
| Peaceful | ◯ ◯ ◯ ◯ ◯ |
| Sleepy | ◯ ◯ ◯ ◯ ◯ |
| Pain Relief | ◯ ◯ ◯ ◯ ◯ |
| Hungry | ◯ ◯ ◯ ◯ ◯ |
| Uplifted | ◯ ◯ ◯ ◯ ◯ |
| Creative | ◯ ◯ ◯ ◯ ◯ |

**Ratings** ☆ ☆ ☆ ☆ ☆

# Strain

Grower

Date

Acquired

$

| Indica | Hybrid | Sativa |
|---|---|---|

- [ ] Flower
- [ ] Edible
- [ ] Concentrate

## Symptoms Relieved

Sweet

Fruity

Floral

Sour

Spicy

Earthy

Herbal

Woodsy

## Notes

| Effects | Strength | | | | |
|---|---|---|---|---|---|
| Peaceful | ○ | ○ | ○ | ○ | ○ |
| Sleepy | ○ | ○ | ○ | ○ | ○ |
| Pain Relief | ○ | ○ | ○ | ○ | ○ |
| Hungry | ○ | ○ | ○ | ○ | ○ |
| Uplifted | ○ | ○ | ○ | ○ | ○ |
| Creative | ○ | ○ | ○ | ○ | ○ |

**Ratings** ☆ ☆ ☆ ☆ ☆

# Strain

Grower

Acquired

Date

$

<table>
<tr><td>Indica</td><td>Hybrid</td><td>Sativa</td></tr>
</table>

☐ Flower  ☐ Edible  ☐ Concentrate

## Symptoms Relieved

## Notes

Sweet · Floral · Spicy · Herbal · Woodsy · Earthy · Sour · Fruity

| Effects | Strength | | | | |
|---|---|---|---|---|---|
| Peaceful | ○ | ○ | ○ | ○ | ○ |
| Sleepy | ○ | ○ | ○ | ○ | ○ |
| Pain Relief | ○ | ○ | ○ | ○ | ○ |
| Hungry | ○ | ○ | ○ | ○ | ○ |
| Uplifted | ○ | ○ | ○ | ○ | ○ |
| Creative | ○ | ○ | ○ | ○ | ○ |

**Ratings** ☆ ☆ ☆ ☆ ☆

# Strain

Grower

Date

Acquired

$

| Indica | Hybrid | Sativa |

☐ Flower  ☐ Edible  ☐ Concentrate

## Symptoms Relieved

Sweet

Fruity

Floral

Sour

Spicy

Earthy

Herbal

Woodsy

## Notes

| Effects | Strength |
| --- | --- |
| Peaceful | ○ ○ ○ ○ ○ |
| Sleepy | ○ ○ ○ ○ ○ |
| Pain Relief | ○ ○ ○ ○ ○ |
| Hungry | ○ ○ ○ ○ ○ |
| Uplifted | ○ ○ ○ ○ ○ |
| Creative | ○ ○ ○ ○ ○ |

**Ratings** ☆ ☆ ☆ ☆ ☆

# Strain

Grower

Date

Acquired

$

| Indica | Hybrid | Sativa |

☐ Flower  ☐ Edible  ☐ Concentrate

## Symptoms Relieved

Sweet

Fruity

Floral

Sour

Spicy

Earthy

Herbal

Woodsy

## Notes

| **Effects** | **Strength** |
| --- | --- |
| Peaceful | ○ ○ ○ ○ ○ |
| Sleepy | ○ ○ ○ ○ ○ |
| Pain Relief | ○ ○ ○ ○ ○ |
| Hungry | ○ ○ ○ ○ ○ |
| Uplifted | ○ ○ ○ ○ ○ |
| Creative | ○ ○ ○ ○ ○ |

**Ratings** ☆ ☆ ☆ ☆ ☆

# Strain

Grower

Date

Acquired

$

| Indica | Hybrid | Sativa |

☐ Flower  ☐ Edible  ☐ Concentrate

## Symptoms Relieved

Sweet

Fruity

Floral

Sour

Spicy

Earthy

Herbal

Woodsy

## Notes

| Effects | Strength |
| --- | --- |
| Peaceful | ○ ○ ○ ○ ○ |
| Sleepy | ○ ○ ○ ○ ○ |
| Pain Relief | ○ ○ ○ ○ ○ |
| Hungry | ○ ○ ○ ○ ○ |
| Uplifted | ○ ○ ○ ○ ○ |
| Creative | ○ ○ ○ ○ ○ |

**Ratings** ☆ ☆ ☆ ☆ ☆

# Strain

Grower

Date

Acquired

$

| Indica | Hybrid | Sativa |

☐ Flower    ☐ Edible    ☐ Concentrate

## Symptoms Relieved

## Notes



| Effects | Strength | | | | |
|---|---|---|---|---|---|
| Peaceful | ○ | ○ | ○ | ○ | ○ |
| Sleepy | ○ | ○ | ○ | ○ | ○ |
| Pain Relief | ○ | ○ | ○ | ○ | ○ |
| Hungry | ○ | ○ | ○ | ○ | ○ |
| Uplifted | ○ | ○ | ○ | ○ | ○ |
| Creative | ○ | ○ | ○ | ○ | ○ |

**Ratings** ☆ ☆ ☆ ☆ ☆

# Strain

Grower

Date

Acquired

$

| Indica | Hybrid | Sativa |
| --- | --- | --- |

☐ Flower    ☐ Edible    ☐ Concentrate

## Symptoms Relieved

## Notes

Sweet

Fruity

Floral

Sour

Spicy

Earthy

Herbal

Woodsy

| Effects | Strength | | | | |
| --- | --- | --- | --- | --- | --- |
| Peaceful | ○ | ○ | ○ | ○ | ○ |
| Sleepy | ○ | ○ | ○ | ○ | ○ |
| Pain Relief | ○ | ○ | ○ | ○ | ○ |
| Hungry | ○ | ○ | ○ | ○ | ○ |
| Uplifted | ○ | ○ | ○ | ○ | ○ |
| Creative | ○ | ○ | ○ | ○ | ○ |

**Ratings** ☆ ☆ ☆ ☆ ☆

# Strain

Grower

Date

Acquired

$

| Indica | Hybrid | Sativa |

☐ Flower   ☐ Edible   ☐ Concentrate

## Symptoms Relieved

## Notes

Sweet
Fruity
Floral
Sour
Spicy
Earthy
Herbal
Woodsy

| Effects | Strength | | | | |
| --- | --- | --- | --- | --- | --- |
| Peaceful | ○ | ○ | ○ | ○ | ○ |
| Sleepy | ○ | ○ | ○ | ○ | ○ |
| Pain Relief | ○ | ○ | ○ | ○ | ○ |
| Hungry | ○ | ○ | ○ | ○ | ○ |
| Uplifted | ○ | ○ | ○ | ○ | ○ |
| Creative | ○ | ○ | ○ | ○ | ○ |

**Ratings** ☆ ☆ ☆ ☆ ☆

# Strain

Grower

Date

Acquired

$

| Indica | Hybrid | Sativa |

☐ Flower   ☐ Edible   ☐ Concentrate

## Symptoms Relieved

Sweet

Fruity

Floral

Sour

Spicy

Earthy

Herbal

Woodsy

## Notes

| Effects | Strength |
|---|---|
| Peaceful | ◯ ◯ ◯ ◯ ◯ |
| Sleepy | ◯ ◯ ◯ ◯ ◯ |
| Pain Relief | ◯ ◯ ◯ ◯ ◯ |
| Hungry | ◯ ◯ ◯ ◯ ◯ |
| Uplifted | ◯ ◯ ◯ ◯ ◯ |
| Creative | ◯ ◯ ◯ ◯ ◯ |

**Ratings** ☆ ☆ ☆ ☆ ☆

# Strain

Grower

Date

Acquired

$

| Indica | Hybrid | Sativa |

☐ Flower ☐ Edible ☐ Concentrate

## Symptoms Relieved

Sweet

Fruity

Floral

Sour

Spicy

Earthy

Herbal

Woodsy

## Notes

| **Effects** | **Strength** |

Peaceful ◯ ◯ ◯ ◯ ◯

Sleepy ◯ ◯ ◯ ◯ ◯

Pain Relief ◯ ◯ ◯ ◯ ◯

Hungry ◯ ◯ ◯ ◯ ◯

Uplifted ◯ ◯ ◯ ◯ ◯

Creative ◯ ◯ ◯ ◯ ◯

**Ratings** ☆ ☆ ☆ ☆ ☆

# Strain

Grower

Acquired

Date

$

|  |  |  |
|---|---|---|
| Indica | Hybrid | Sativa |

☐ Flower   ☐ Edible   ☐ Concentrate

## Symptoms Relieved

Sweet
Fruity
Floral
Sour
Spicy
Earthy
Herbal
Woodsy

## Notes

| Effects | Strength | | | | |
|---|---|---|---|---|---|
| Peaceful | ○ | ○ | ○ | ○ | ○ |
| Sleepy | ○ | ○ | ○ | ○ | ○ |
| Pain Relief | ○ | ○ | ○ | ○ | ○ |
| Hungry | ○ | ○ | ○ | ○ | ○ |
| Uplifted | ○ | ○ | ○ | ○ | ○ |
| Creative | ○ | ○ | ○ | ○ | ○ |

**Ratings** ☆ ☆ ☆ ☆ ☆

# Strain

Grower

Date

Acquired

$

| Indica | Hybrid | Sativa |

☐ Flower  ☐ Edible  ☐ Concentrate

## Symptoms Relieved

Sweet

Fruity

Floral

Sour

Spicy

Earthy

Herbal

Woodsy

## Notes

| **Effects** | | **Strength** | | |
| --- | --- | --- | --- | --- |
| Peaceful | ○ | ○ | ○ | ○ | ○ |
| Sleepy | ○ | ○ | ○ | ○ | ○ |
| Pain Relief | ○ | ○ | ○ | ○ | ○ |
| Hungry | ○ | ○ | ○ | ○ | ○ |
| Uplifted | ○ | ○ | ○ | ○ | ○ |
| Creative | ○ | ○ | ○ | ○ | ○ |

**Ratings** ☆ ☆ ☆ ☆ ☆

# Strain

Grower

Date

Acquired

$

| Indica | Hybrid | Sativa |

☐ Flower　　☐ Edible　　☐ Concentrate

## Symptoms Relieved

## Notes



| Effects | Strength |
| --- | --- |
| Peaceful | ○ ○ ○ ○ ○ |
| Sleepy | ○ ○ ○ ○ ○ |
| Pain Relief | ○ ○ ○ ○ ○ |
| Hungry | ○ ○ ○ ○ ○ |
| Uplifted | ○ ○ ○ ○ ○ |
| Creative | ○ ○ ○ ○ ○ |

**Ratings** ☆ ☆ ☆ ☆ ☆

# Strain

Grower

Date

Acquired

$

| Indica | Hybrid | Sativa |

☐ Flower     ☐ Edible     ☐ Concentrate

## Symptoms Relieved

Sweet
Fruity
Floral
Sour
Spicy
Earthy
Herbal
Woodsy

## Notes

| Effects | Strength |
| --- | --- |
| Peaceful | ○ ○ ○ ○ ○ |
| Sleepy | ○ ○ ○ ○ ○ |
| Pain Relief | ○ ○ ○ ○ ○ |
| Hungry | ○ ○ ○ ○ ○ |
| Uplifted | ○ ○ ○ ○ ○ |
| Creative | ○ ○ ○ ○ ○ |

**Ratings** ☆ ☆ ☆ ☆ ☆

# Strain

Grower ___________________ Date ___________________

Acquired ___________________ $ ___________________

| Indica | Hybrid | Sativa |
|:---:|:---:|:---:|

☐ Flower ☐ Edible ☐ Concentrate

## Symptoms Relieved

## Notes

Sweet
Fruity
Floral
Sour
Spicy
Earthy
Herbal
Woodsy

| Effects | Strength | | | | |
|---|---|---|---|---|---|
| Peaceful | ○ | ○ | ○ | ○ | ○ |
| Sleepy | ○ | ○ | ○ | ○ | ○ |
| Pain Relief | ○ | ○ | ○ | ○ | ○ |
| Hungry | ○ | ○ | ○ | ○ | ○ |
| Uplifted | ○ | ○ | ○ | ○ | ○ |
| Creative | ○ | ○ | ○ | ○ | ○ |

**Ratings** ☆ ☆ ☆ ☆ ☆

# Strain

Grower

Date

Acquired

$

| Indica | Hybrid | Sativa |

☐ Flower   ☐ Edible   ☐ Concentrate

## Symptoms Relieved



## Notes

| **Effects** | **Strength** | | | | |
|---|---|---|---|---|---|
| Peaceful | ○ | ○ | ○ | ○ | ○ |
| Sleepy | ○ | ○ | ○ | ○ | ○ |
| Pain Relief | ○ | ○ | ○ | ○ | ○ |
| Hungry | ○ | ○ | ○ | ○ | ○ |
| Uplifted | ○ | ○ | ○ | ○ | ○ |
| Creative | ○ | ○ | ○ | ○ | ○ |

**Ratings** ☆ ☆ ☆ ☆ ☆

# Strain

Grower

Date

Acquired

$

| Indica | Hybrid | Sativa |

☐ Flower  ☐ Edible  ☐ Concentrate

## Symptoms Relieved

Sweet

Fruity

Floral

Sour

Spicy

Earthy

Herbal

Woodsy

## Notes

| **Effects** | **Strength** |

Peaceful ○ ○ ○ ○ ○

Sleepy ○ ○ ○ ○ ○

Pain Relief ○ ○ ○ ○ ○

Hungry ○ ○ ○ ○ ○

Uplifted ○ ○ ○ ○ ○

Creative ○ ○ ○ ○ ○

**Ratings** ☆ ☆ ☆ ☆ ☆

# Strain

Grower

Date

Acquired

$

| Indica | Hybrid | Sativa |
|---|---|---|

☐ Flower  ☐ Edible  ☐ Concentrate

## Symptoms Relieved

Sweet
Fruity
Floral
Sour
Spicy
Earthy
Herbal
Woodsy

## Notes

| Effects | Strength | | | | |
|---|---|---|---|---|---|
| Peaceful | ○ | ○ | ○ | ○ | ○ |
| Sleepy | ○ | ○ | ○ | ○ | ○ |
| Pain Relief | ○ | ○ | ○ | ○ | ○ |
| Hungry | ○ | ○ | ○ | ○ | ○ |
| Uplifted | ○ | ○ | ○ | ○ | ○ |
| Creative | ○ | ○ | ○ | ○ | ○ |

**Ratings** ☆ ☆ ☆ ☆ ☆

# Strain

Grower

Date

Acquired

$

| Indica | Hybrid | Sativa |

☐ Flower    ☐ Edible    ☐ Concentrate

## Symptoms Relieved



## Notes

| Effects | Strength |
| --- | --- |
| Peaceful | ○ ○ ○ ○ ○ |
| Sleepy | ○ ○ ○ ○ ○ |
| Pain Relief | ○ ○ ○ ○ ○ |
| Hungry | ○ ○ ○ ○ ○ |
| Uplifted | ○ ○ ○ ○ ○ |
| Creative | ○ ○ ○ ○ ○ |

**Ratings** ☆ ☆ ☆ ☆ ☆

# Strain

Grower

Date

Acquired

$

| Indica | Hybrid | Sativa |

☐ Flower  ☐ Edible  ☐ Concentrate

## Symptoms Relieved



## Notes

| Effects | Strength |
| --- | --- |
| Peaceful | ○ ○ ○ ○ ○ |
| Sleepy | ○ ○ ○ ○ ○ |
| Pain Relief | ○ ○ ○ ○ ○ |
| Hungry | ○ ○ ○ ○ ○ |
| Uplifted | ○ ○ ○ ○ ○ |
| Creative | ○ ○ ○ ○ ○ |

**Ratings** ☆ ☆ ☆ ☆ ☆

# Strain

Grower

Date

Acquired

$

| Indica | Hybrid | Sativa |

☐ Flower  ☐ Edible  ☐ Concentrate

## Symptoms Relieved



## Notes

| Effects | Strength |
| --- | --- |
| Peaceful | ◯ ◯ ◯ ◯ ◯ |
| Sleepy | ◯ ◯ ◯ ◯ ◯ |
| Pain Relief | ◯ ◯ ◯ ◯ ◯ |
| Hungry | ◯ ◯ ◯ ◯ ◯ |
| Uplifted | ◯ ◯ ◯ ◯ ◯ |
| Creative | ◯ ◯ ◯ ◯ ◯ |

**Ratings** ☆ ☆ ☆ ☆ ☆

# Strain

Grower

Date

Acquired

$

| Indica | Hybrid | Sativa |
| --- | --- | --- |

☐ Flower  ☐ Edible  ☐ Concentrate

## Symptoms Relieved

Sweet

Fruity

Floral

Sour

Spicy

Earthy

Herbal

Woodsy

## Notes

| Effects | Strength | | | | |
| --- | --- | --- | --- | --- | --- |
| Peaceful | ○ | ○ | ○ | ○ | ○ |
| Sleepy | ○ | ○ | ○ | ○ | ○ |
| Pain Relief | ○ | ○ | ○ | ○ | ○ |
| Hungry | ○ | ○ | ○ | ○ | ○ |
| Uplifted | ○ | ○ | ○ | ○ | ○ |
| Creative | ○ | ○ | ○ | ○ | ○ |

**Ratings** ☆ ☆ ☆ ☆ ☆

# Strain

Grower

Date

Acquired

$

| Indica | Hybrid | Sativa |

☐ Flower    ☐ Edible    ☐ Concentrate

## Symptoms Relieved

Sweet

Fruity

Floral

Sour

Spicy

Earthy

Herbal

Woodsy

## Notes

| Effects | Strength |
| --- | --- |
| Peaceful | ○ ○ ○ ○ ○ |
| Sleepy | ○ ○ ○ ○ ○ |
| Pain Relief | ○ ○ ○ ○ ○ |
| Hungry | ○ ○ ○ ○ ○ |
| Uplifted | ○ ○ ○ ○ ○ |
| Creative | ○ ○ ○ ○ ○ |

**Ratings** ☆ ☆ ☆ ☆ ☆

# Strain

Grower

Date

Acquired

$

| Indica | Hybrid | Sativa |

☐ Flower  ☐ Edible  ☐ Concentrate

## Symptoms Relieved

## Notes

Sweet

Fruity

Floral

Sour

Spicy

Earthy

Herbal

Woodsy

| Effects | Strength |
|---|---|
| Peaceful | ○ ○ ○ ○ ○ |
| Sleepy | ○ ○ ○ ○ ○ |
| Pain Relief | ○ ○ ○ ○ ○ |
| Hungry | ○ ○ ○ ○ ○ |
| Uplifted | ○ ○ ○ ○ ○ |
| Creative | ○ ○ ○ ○ ○ |

**Ratings** ☆ ☆ ☆ ☆ ☆

Made in the USA
Monee, IL
07 July 2026